M000026102

NATURAL THERAPIES FOR AUTISM: UPDATES ON THE RESEARCH

(for practitioners and parents)

by Dan Purser MD

www.drpursernaturaloptions.com

Copyright © 2015 by Dan Purser MD.

All Rights Reserved.

No part of this publication may be reproduced, distributed, or transmitted in any form or by any means, including photocopying, recording, or other electronic or mechanical methods, or by any information storage and retrieval system without the prior written permission of the publisher, except in the case of very brief quotations embodied in critical reviews and certain other noncommercial uses permitted by copyright law.

Get more Kindle health series books here: GreatMedEbooks.com Published by DP Publishing LLC.

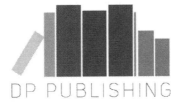

DP PUBLISHING

My Legal Protection

Do not use the information contained in this book to treat yourself or your child. Please consult with a knowledgeable physician in your area before starting any treatment as might possibly be suggested in this book. I will not be held responsible if something goes wrong. So BE CAREFUL!

Thank you.

Table of Contents

FOREWORD

This little book arose from a talk I first gave at a Young Living Essential Oil Thrive™ event in Nashville, Tennessee in February of 2015. The Thrive™ event, attended by over 3,000 women (and some men), was sponsored by a wonderful lady and her husband, top distributors for Young Living™ Essential Oils, named Monique and Jeremiah McLean. So in a way, that talk, and now this book is their doing. They're great parents and genuinely nice people – and well loved – as are their children, I'm sure, but this talk caused a little bit of a firestorm as it came out of the blue, was totally unexpected and much talked about in natural circles afterwards.

So I dedicate this book to Monique and Jeremiah McLean and their children, my awesome son, and all the children out there who are special and better than most in so many ways, including those of the Autism Spectrum Disorder and it's derivatives, and to their long suffering and loving parents – I hope it sheds some small light on a sometimes dark and winding path for them all.

Autism is a neurological disorder. It's not caused by bad parenting. It's caused by, you know, abnormal development in the brain. The emotional circuits in the brain are abnormal. And there also are differences in the white matter, which is the brain's computer cables that hook up the different brain departments.
--Temple Grandin

CHAPTER 1

CAUSES OF AUTISM

Brain Health = Child Health

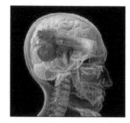 

DAN PURSER MD

I don't see many patients each day – I try to keep the number below eight. I know some of my doctor colleagues see over 50-60 patients, on average, a day. That's great, for them, but maybe I'm slow or something. I like to really dive deep with each patient and then look at the root cause of their issues. I never do "bandaids" – just not in my wheelhouse. So I spend a lot of time taking detailed histories. Labs, medications, and vitamins are also thoroughly reviewed – no stone unturned. I also really enjoy going home and spending time with my family, my children, wife and some other fun projects – probably why I've had ten #1 books on Amazon as I write this.

That's what this book is about – diving deeper, my way, into autism. So let's start.

I believe anything you can do for the brain to be healthy, or healthier, will help the entire body –

especially the child's body – YOUR child's body to be healthier, more sound and last longer.

Autism has been thought to have been caused by many different things over the years but in this little book I wish to redefine it to what experts and researchers are out there talking about – talking about today – in 2015 – about what the current research is telling us about how it should be defined, and why it occurs.

First – it's clear that autism is incredibly complex – much more diverse and intricate than originally thought to be.

Second, the causes of ASD (Autism Spectrum Disorder) are incredibly multifactorial in nature, so we have to accept that.

Third, and on the other hand, ASD's has received few universal truths about it that are falling into place – common denominators that cannot be denied. And that has to be addressed. So I'll try to address those too.

Fourth, the research into natural options, therapies and cures is surprisingly sparse – which should be bothersome to parents of autistic children as there are literally millions of kids not growing up and aging with autism – a massive wall of them in the state in which I live – Utah.

So I'll try to define those causes better so in the future we have no more walls of kids with autism rolling towards us – that we slow the growth of this nightmare down – and then we can look at what can be done for young adults or children with autism or ASD.

My Past Beliefs on Causes of ASD

I'm a physician, researcher, author, and parent with 30 years experience – and I had mixed ideas in my head about autism – something vague as to the causation – heavy metal storage problem? Or something. I had no clearly defined beliefs, really.

That changed about five years ago when I became involved with a new form of glutathione that no one had ever seen before – it was topical, stable, reduced, and complexed into a sugar molecule (to protect from oxidation) – really the only way, the only form, that glutathione could realistically be absorbed and used by the body (more on this later). One of our pituitary endocrinology teammates had created it (outside of the university) when I was doing research in southern California, and these guys all taught at USC's Kleck School of Medicine – the one who actually came up with it teaches a nanotechnology course at USC and is a PhD pharmacologist. He said he'd developed it specifically for the treatment of kids with autism. It was a definite "Ahah! Moment" for me as I started looking at this form of glutathione and how it could be used. I was amazed and overwhelmed.

I also had my own family member with what we'd thought was mild ASD (we'd come to that conclusion after this person reached adulthood though and felt there was nothing that could be done). So it impacted me personally and in a big way.

Preparing for Thrive™ in Nashville 2015

My view of autism took another sea change on me as I was preparing to speak at the Young Living™ Essential Oils sponsored Thrive™ event in Nashville in February of 2015 – there'd be an estimated 3,000 women in attendance. Monique McLean and her husband had asked that I speak at the last minute when another physician had a severe medical emergency – at this point in my life I'd probably spoken in front of even larger crowds dozens of times so it was nothing new but usually I spoke about hormones and endocrinology (since I did research in that area). I'd also had 5 of my books be #1 at least 7 times in 10 different categories on Amazon™. The trouble I was having as I prepared was that I had three time blocks to cover – so I'd do women's hormones, men's hormones and what?

I couldn't decide.

I'd recently been asked to be the medical director of the Utah State Developmental Center in American Fork, Utah and was struggling with taking on the position as my plate was quite full. The director, Guy Thompson (a great guy, by the way, in a very difficult job) had told me they were expecting a wall of young adults with autism (and ASD) to soon be enrolling in the facility because their individual communities had neither the resources nor the ability to handle them and so they needed my help as a medical director – it was pretty far from my day job, where I work in a plastic surgery group dealing with complex wound issues (on top of many, many other things – I own seven successful companies). His comments had also caused me to start looking up research on ASD and what was being done out there. I'd been a little surprised at my findings.

I'd discovered many interesting things about autism and ASD and the causes.

In the end, my third block talk at Thrive™ (and this book) was a report on those findings and the treatments for those issues (if there is one) – one of which is just a natural conclusion to the problem noted – and what I said in Nashville that day that had so many mom's asking for this book.

What I Found in the Research

People have known for years that autism had to be something genetic but in 1998 a doctor (a neurologist named Jay Lombard, MD) at Westchester Square Medical Center in New York hypothesized in the June edition of the journal MEDICAL HYPOTHESES that autism and ASD appeared quite similar to other mitochondrial dysfunction disorders.

Why did he say this?

Mitochondrial dysfunction disorders have the same awkward movement and similar speech and cognitive patterns as ASD.

First -- what is a mitochondria?

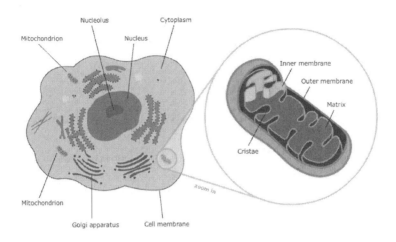

It is the powerhouse of the cell. It is the small oval or pill shaped structure within our cells (usually thousands of these are in each cell).

What does it mean to be the powerhouse of the cell?

The human body cannot directly use sugar as an energy source so we must convert the sugar into ATP (adenosine triphosphate), which our cells can directly use. This conversion of sugar to ATP occurs in the mitochondria utilizing the aerobic pathway consisting of Glycolysis, the Citric Acid Cycle (some call it the Kreb's Cycle) and finally the Electron Transport Chain are all contained in the mitochondria.

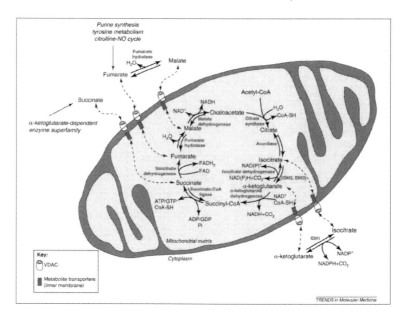

Confused? Don't be – just hang in there.

So what are the main duties of the mitochondria?

(Following list is from http://www.ivyroses.com/Biology/Organelles/Function -of-Mitochondria.php)

1. Production of energy

ATP Synthesis

The main function of mitochondria is the production of ATP.

According to many textbooks: Energy production within cells is the main function of mitochondria. However, some students are told not to state that mitochondria "produce" or "create" energy. Strictly, the energy is released from storage (in chemical bonds) by reactions that occur in mitochondria. According to the Law of Conservation of Energy, the total amount of energy in an isolated system remains constant over time. A-Level Biology students can say that mitochondria are the site of aerobic respiration in eukaryotic cells.

This occurs by a process of cellular respiration, also known as aerobic respiration, which is dependent on the presence of oxygen. (When oxygen is limited, the chemicals that would otherwise be oxidized are, instead, metabolized by anaerobic respiration, via a process that is independent of the mitochondria.)

The 3 main stages in the overall process of aerobic cellular respiration are:

A. Glycolysis -- splitting sugar molecules

B. TCA Cycle -- The tricarboxylic acid cycle (TCA cycle) is a series of enzyme-catalyzed chemical reactions that form a key part of aerobic respiration in cells. This cycle is also called the Krebs Cycle and/or the citric acid cycle.

C. Electron Transport -- An electron transport chain (ETC) is a series of compounds that transfer electrons from electron donors to electron acceptors via redox reactions, and couples this electron transfer with the transfer of protons (H+ ions) across a membrane.

2. Production of heat

Non-shivering thermogenesis

The term thermogenesis refers to heat production in living organisms, mainly mammals. It is classified according to how the heat production is initiated:

Exercise-associated thermogenesis - due to movement e.g. shivering.

Non-exercise activity thermogenesis - incl. non-shivering thermogenesis,
see below.

Diet-induced thermogenesis - i.e. heat generated by the body following the digestive processes. See also metabolic rate.

Non-shivering thermogenesis is due to facilitated diffusion of protons into the mitochondrial matrix. This is called "proton leak" or "mitochondrial uncoupling" and only occurs in certain circumstances. When it does happen, this results in the unharnessed potential energy of the proton electrochemical gradient being released as heat.

Non-shivering thermogenesis occurs mainly in brown adipose tissue, also known as "brown fat" (adipose tissue is "fat tissue") because the process is controlled by a protein present in brown fat. The protein is thermogenin, also known as UCP1, and acts as a proton channel that sometimes enables protons (i.e. $H+$ ions) to enter the mitochondrial matrix without contributing to ATP synthesis.

Brown adipose tissue is produced in various amounts by different types of mammals and is at its highest levels in early life and in hibernating animals e.g. bears living in cold environments. Adult humans usually only have small brown fat deposits throughout the body - brown fat is present in humans at birth, but decreases with age.

3. Role as independent units within eukaryotic cells

Mitochondria have mitochondrial DNA (mtDNA). Mitochondria are really cells within cells so this only makes sense – they are part of the jigsaw of the elegant design we underwent in our history.

Mitochondria contain their own genetic material - which is independent of the cell in which they are located – and this always comes from the mother.

So mitochondrial DNA (mtDNA) is maternally inherited. At fertilization only nuclear DNA enters from the sperm because although the egg contains mitochondria, sperm cells do not. Sperm are so tiny that mitochondria would hamper their passage toward the egg. (Therefore exercise capacity e.g. for endurance sports tends to be maternally inherited. Maternal ancestral history can also be traced via mtDNA.)

mtDNA accounts for about 1% of the total cellular DNA - recall that the number of mitochondria per cell varies considerably with the type and function of the cell. mtDNA exists in a circular arrangement in the mitochondrial matrix. Mutations of errors in some mitochondrial genes can result in certain diseases - mitochondrial diseases. Mitochondria self-replicate (divide) by fission, as is also true of bacteria cells - which are also known as prokaryotic cells.

4. Role in the process of apoptosis: (Programmed cell death)

Two types of cell death occur in multicellular organisms:

Apoptosis - the process of programmed cell death (PCD), in which biochemical changes lead to cell changes such as cell shrinkage, nuclear fragmentation, chromatin condensation, and chromosomal DNA fragmentation, the ultimate consequence of which is death of the cell.

Necrosis - traumatic (not pre-planned or "programmed") cell death e.g. due to acute cellular injury.

Apoptosis is advantageous to organisms for many reasons. For example, during development it is necessary for some cells to die in order for normal tissue and organ formation to proceed, e.g. the differentiation of fingers in a human embryo occurs by apoptosis of the cells between the fingers, resulting in separate fingers. Death of abnormal cells such as cells that are cancerous or virally infected is also good for the organism. Unlike necrosis, apoptosis results in cell fragments called apoptotic bodies that phagocytic cells can engulf and quickly remove before the contents of the cell spills over surrounding cells which could cause tissue damage.

Mitochondria help to safeguard cell survival while appropriate and to facilitate apoptosis when necessary. When apoptosis of a cell is stimulated: pro-apoptotic proteins insert into the mitochondrial membrane, forming pores in the membrane.

Pro-apoptotic proteins insert into the mitochondrial membrane, forming pores in the membrane.

A protein called cytochrome leaves the intermembrane space of the mitochondrion via the pores in the mitochondrial membrane.

Cytochrome emerges from the mitochondrion into the cytosol (i.e. the intracellular fluid) of the eukaryotic cell – of our healthy cells.

Cytochrome in the cytosol of the cell stimulates a cascade of biochemical changes that lead to apoptotic death of the cell and this death is really critical as you can't have a lot of worthless dysfunctional scruddy cells sitting doing nothing but absorbing energy – the human body would last about 7-10 years at most – we'd have all ended before we started way back when.

5. Storage of Ca2+ ions

Calcium (Ca2+) has many important functions in the biochemistry of cells and in physiology generally, e.g.r.e.

1. signal transduction pathways
2. neurotransmitter release from neurons
3. contraction of muscle cells
4. many enzymes need Ca2+ as a cofactor, e.g. in blood-clotting
5. fertilization
6. ... and extracellular calcium is needed to maintain the potential difference across excitable cell membranes, and for the formation of healthy bones

Storage of Calcium (Ca2+):

In the case of mammals, including humans, bone tissue is the main mineral storage site. Release and re-absorption of Ca2+ from and into bone is regulated by hormones. At a cellular level, Ca2+ is held within two types of organelles, the endoplasmic reticulum and mitochondria. The endoplasmic reticulum (SER & RER) is the main site of cellular storage of calcium. Mitochondria can also transiently store calcium - contributing to the cell's homeostasis of calcium by acting as "cytosolic buffers" for calcium.

6. **Other mitochondrial functions include the following:[i]**

- Building, breakdown, and recycling of products that are needed for the cell to function normally
- Formation of parts of blood and hormones such as estrogen and testosterone
- Synthesis of steroids
- Regulation of membrane potential
- Monitoring of cell differentiation, growth, and development
- Cell signaling of neurons

Let's Look At The List Again

1. **Production of energy**
2. **Production of heat**
3. **Role as independent units within eukaryotic cells**
4. **Role in the process of apoptosis: (Programmed cell death)**
5. **Storage of Ca2+ ions**
6. **Other mitochondrial functions (i.e. hormones)**

Now ponder issues that children with ASD have and compare them to this list – they have trouble with energy, they get tired easily, they have low hormones (at least the ASD children I've checked), they have osteoporosis issues and can tend to be quite frail, and they have difficulty clearing toxins.

Hmmm, sounds like mitochondrial dysfunction is a good possibility.

But The Most Important Mitochondrial Function (In My Opinion) Is...

But the most important function, for the sake of this discussion, is removing toxic dead cells.

Mitochondria kill damaged cells!

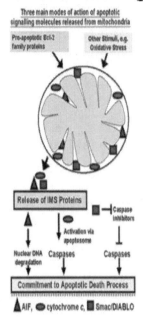

CHAPTER 2

MTHFR AND UNDERMETHYLATION CONDITIONS

An Interesting Root Cause Defect

The vast majority of children with the Spectrum (ASD) can't make glutathione – or more appropriately cannot make the enzyme, glutathione peroxidase (GPX), that removes the toxin or oxidants off of the oxidized glutathione (GSSG) in order to make it into a functional version of glutathione – GSH (a lot more on this later).

What could cause this lack of GPX? It's a genetic problem – it has to be. There are reasonably no other options. And it's probably more than one genetic malfunction.

But whenever I do intracellular vitamin and mineral levels on children in the Autism Spectrum, or on adults who appear to have ASD, I keep getting low intracellular GSH levels (to be expected) along with low intracellular levels of B12 and pantothenate. Most bad MTHFR cases cannot make GPX meaning they cannot make reduced glutathione (GSH).

This combination indicates only one thing to me – MTHFR. Usually homozygous bad MTHFR (homozygous means you have two gene mutations). Now not all people with MTHFR snps (gene mutations) have the chemical problems or diseases associated with MTHFR – but if someone has the symptoms there are some tests I highly advise to pursue this genetic condition – and these can REALLY help your child with autism or ASD.

TESTS for MTHFR (and ASD)

- o Spectracell Comprehensive Micronutrient Panel
- o Spcetracell MTHFR Genetic Testing
- o Serum Homocysteine Level
- o Whole Blood Histamine Level

Later I discuss the Spectracell Micronutrient Panel and how it looks at 39 different INTRACELLULAR vitamins and minerals – IMHO, it is the best test on the planet for kids with autism or ASD. For heaven's sakes – you're looking at intracellular levels – that is crazy technology and is earthshattering for kids with autism. It lets you look under the hood in a way no other test can.

Usually the test will show your child has trouble handling certain B vitamins at a cellular level. It can also show a depressed intracellular glutathione level (another problem caused by MTHFR genetic problems and common in autism). That indicates all MTHFR snps are indeed impacting cellular health.

Please keep in mind this is an incredibly complex set of interactions – as people tend to have many different little snps and mutations (if patients are incredibly curious about this I advise the 23andme testing which is cheap ($99) and very detailed and easy to do – just spit into the tubes – I know GROSS but still...) and the possible problems or interactions can be mind numbing. But the main thing you worry about in this situation is the impact MTHFR might have on your child's intracellular levels and enzymes and certain substances – studies have shown that most kids (98%) with ASD have MTHFR snps[ii] and more, are histamine "undermethylators"!

Want to know more about this? You need to get a handle on this – this is complicated stuff – get a book on MTHFR (any book or at least my book called **THE 85% SOLUTION** which has protocols and research in it – yes, there's LOTS of research on MTHFR while not on autism or ASD). Also watch this video by Dr Mensah on "Mental Health and MTHFR SNPS"[iii] and also this excellent blog post on methylation by Dr. Judy Tsafrir.[iv] The following is lifted directly from that book I wrote.

FIRST -- Defining Under- and Over- Methylators

Let's say your whole blood histamine level is 90 ng/ml (or high – according to the results of your local lab). According to Dr William Walsh (in his bestselling book "Nutrient Power: Heal Your Biochemistry and Heal Your Brain" by William J. Walsh, PhD) an optimal histamine range is 25-65 ng/ml or 40-70 ng/ml (according to which lab you use), thereby classifying someone who's higher than 70 as an "Undermethylator".

An Undermethylator is intolerant to folate because it lowers serotonin even more, making them more depressed.

Methylfolate Causes Cancer? What?

There is a common misconception, however, that the mere presence of an MTHFR mutation is synonymous with a methylation defect. This is by no means necessarily the case, even if an individual is homozygous for the gene. The presence of the defective gene does not necessarily translate into a functional defect. In fact, the recent wide spread indiscriminate prescription of methylfolate to compensate for the genetic mutation is not only misguided, but can actually make people who are undermethylated not only feel much worse, but also increase their risk of developing cancer.[v]

So How Do You Figure This Out?

In order to determine the actual functional methylation status in the body, whole blood histamine must be measured. Histamine levels correlate with the functionality of the methylation process. Histamine and methyl are inversely related to one another. That is to say, if whole blood histamine is low, the individual will be overmethylated and if it is high, they will be undermethylated.

The protocols to treat the two conditions are different.[vi]

So What Causes Histamine Intolerance?

Common causes include:[vii]

- Inflammatory bowel diseases (or anything that causes damage to the enterocytes -the cells that line the gut)
- Celiac disease
- Intestinal dysbiosis
- Small Intestinal Bacterial Overgrowth (SIBO)
- Parasitic infections, like Giardia
- Leaky gut or increase in intestinal permeability
- Alcohol or other DAO inhibitors
- Excess biogenic amines in diet
- Medications that increase histamine
- Food allergies
- Genetic polymorphisms, like MTHFR and others that lower DAO, MAO, ALDH
- Vitamin cofactor deficiencies - enzymes, like DAO and MAO rely on vitamin co-factors and deficiencies these can also cause abnormal enzyme activity."

Too Much Folate Causes Depression? Really?

- "A wide range of abnormal chemistries and behaviors were observed in the depressive population.

- 5 chemical classifications (phenotypes) were identified, representing 95% of depressives.

- Distinctive symptoms and traits were identified for each depression group.

Chemical Classification of Depression[viii]

- 38% Undermethylation
- 20% Folate Deficiency
- 17% Copper Overload
- 15% Elevated Pyrroles
- 5% Toxic Metal Overload

Implications of Database Findings on Depression[ix]

- Depression is a name given to a variety of different mood disorders.

- Each depression phenotype has unique chemical imbalances and symptoms.

- Different treatment approaches are needed for these disorders.

A 25-Year Mystery Solved![x]

- Folic Acid is a very-effective methylating agent.

- Undermethylated depressed patients (HIGH Histamine Level) are intolerant to folates.

- Overmethylated depressives (LOW Histamine Level) thrive on folates.

WHY?

Serotonin Mystery Solved by Epigenetic Science[xi]

- Folic Acid generates acetylase enzymes that alter histones & promote expression of SERT (SERT = serotonin transporter).

- SERT increases serotonin reuptake, thus reducing serotonin activity.

- For low-serotonin depressives, the harmful impact of folic acid at the synapse exceeds the benefits of normalizing methylation.

Epigenetics of Methyl and Folate[xii]

- SAMe modifies histones to block production of transporter proteins: This reuptake inhibition increases activity of serotonin & dopamine.

- Folates have the opposite effect on histones and lower serotonin and dopamine activity.

Facts About Methylation

Methylation is the act of a carbon and three hydrogens (namely a methyl group) attaching itself to an enzyme in your body. When this methyl group attaches to an enzyme, the enzyme performs a specific action. One thing you might not realize is that methylation is responsible for is the breakdown of histamine. A methyl group is made and then floats around until it finds a specific binding site. In this case, the methyl group binds to histamine. When a methyl group binds to histamine, histamine breaks apart and goes away. Many patients who have one or more methylation SNPs, like MTHFR have a hard time breaking down histamine, which can wreak havoc on the body in many ways[xiii].

When it comes to methylation -- you either don't make enough, make too much, or make just the right amount. And be cautious with the use of folate/folic acid if you are an Undermethylator. Folate is a serotonin reuptake promoter, (antidepressants [SSRI's] are reuptake inhibitors and undermethylated persons respond well to these medications) so its affect on your epigenetic structure will make you feel worse.

Plus, we already talked about this but just because you have the MTHFR genes, this does not mean that they are expressing. There are many epigentic reasons for turning them on and off.

In my opinion it would be very dangerous for anyone to tell a patient to take folate/folic acid if they don't know their methylation status (under-, normal, or over-).

Some symptoms and traits of undermethylation:[xiv]

Chronic depression, history of perfectionism, seasonal allergies, history of oppositional defiance, high libido, adverse reaction to benzodiazepines and folic acid, good response to SSRI's and anti-histamines, sparse body hair, suicidal tendencies, addictiveness, phobias, denial of illness, obsessive compulsive tendencies, ritualistic behaviors, strong willed, self-motivated during school years, history of competitiveness in sports, strong willed, calm demeanor but high inner tension, family history of high accomplishment, frequent headaches, slenderness, dietary inflexibility, terse speech

Some symptoms and traits of overmethylation:[xv]

High anxiety/panic, hyperactivity, rapid speech, low libido, religiosity, tendency to be overweight, nervous legs, pacing, adverse reaction to SSRI's and SAMe, improvement with benzodiazepines, dry eyes and mouth, low motivation during school years, depression, self mutilation, sleep disorder, tinnitus, hirsutism, food/chemical sensitivities, artistic or musical ability, copper overload, estrogen and antihistamine intolerance, absence of seasonal allergies

SAMe Supplementation – Is It Right?

Another aspect is that SAMe is great for an Undermethylator but can cause suicidal/homicidal tendencies in an Overmethylator because their serotonin levels are already elevated.

So you should incorporate histamine testing in your labs for your MTHFR testing.
Because then a "depressed person with MTHFR SNPs" wouldn't become more depressed by taking folate/folic acid and an "overmethylator person with the MTHFR SNPs wouldn't become suicidal by mistakenly taking SAMe.

SOMEONE WHO TOOK SAMe

Let's look at a blog post by someone who took SAMe – THIS IS VERY INFORMATIVE.

BLOG POST FROM PGEN PARTICIPANT[xvi]

"Trying Out SAMe (Smart People Can Do Dumb Things)

First off, it turns out that methylfolate helps people make their OWN SAM-e! They are part of the same cycle, and SAM-e is one of the by-products from MTHFR processing. Regarding taking both, there was virtually no solid evidence floating up to the top, but an awful lot of opinion and personal experience. (Guess I'm adding to that body of unclear literature.) I saw a lot of people saying, "If you have MTHFR deficiency, do not ever take SAMe!" This was balanced by an equal number of folk saying the opposite. The overall picture was unclear. There was a lot that said to take them together, almost nothing about if you have an MTHFR deficiency.

I found one woman who described it as helpful for brief periods, and she described her genetics as similar to mine — heterozygous MTHFR, homozygous COMT (H62H & V158M), and celiac. She described reacting with an over-methylation response after a couple weeks, and I had gone through that when I started taking methylfolate and felt I know what to do. Just to be careful, I started out with the smallest dose I could find – 200mg.

WHAT HAPPENED

Part of what was motivating this was that general feeling of being unwell that I've had ever since I returned from my trip. I really want to feel better, but am feeling crummy. I thought about waiting to start SAMe until I feel better, but based on what information I'd found I thought I knew what to expect. Either it wouldn't do much, or I'd feel better.

I took a half dose on Monday. I felt basically the same as I've been feeling — generally crummy. Tuesday the same thing. I wasn't sure if I'd been glutened or not. I took a couple days off, just to see. Then I thought maybe I hadn't taken enough to notice a difference. [The problem with this was I had forgotten to look at how long it takes to feel an effect, and it varies depending on the problem.]

I was taking Friday as vacation, and thought I'd risk taking a larger dose, since I didn't want to experiment if I was going to try to work. Instead of 200, I took 400. I continued to feel vaguely crummy, and then I started to feel as if I'd been glutened. I'd been eating "whole foods," so I couldn't imagine what it would have been, but I recognized the feeling. Fatigue. Brain fog. Wobbly. But not a hint of any digestive symptoms, no bloating, no hives. I was puzzled, but sleeping too much to figure it out. I had trouble sitting and standing, my joints hurt. I felt too weak to do much. Not normal symptoms included feeling hot, sweaty, feverish, flushed, confused, congested, chilling, spaced out, distractible. Then I got a headache, and my head feels strange in the back. So far, this has lasted three days. Each day has had a couple brief periods when I felt ok, before it would start up again, slightly milder than the day before.

WHAT I LEARNED AFTERWARDS

I went back and looked again at SAMe overdose. Nope, these symptoms don't match up, except for the headache. My symptoms were more like those indicators that someone needs more SAMe. Very puzzling. I kept digging into literature about SAM-e. I tried taking extra methylfolate, but didn't notice a difference. I did notice that my clear-headed time was in late afternoon, and every day I take a B-complex vitamin with my lunch. Then I stumbled into some information that SAM-e can cause problems if someone is deficient in B-vitamins (like me). Basically, it creates a lot of homocysteine, which the body can't clear out because it needs more B-vitamins to do so."

DETAILS: THE FUNCTION OF SAMe

"What is the function of SAMe? The function of SAMe is to simply take what is called a 'methyl group' and give it away to over 200 enzymes in the body in order to perform various critical functions. Some key functions of this freely donated methyl group are to:

Protect your DNA. This is very important. For example, if your DNA is not protected, then it is susceptible to damage by viruses, bacteria, heavy metals, solvents and others. Over time, this damage becomes significant and may result in cancerous cell proliferation.

Reduces histamine levels! Repeating this so it sinks in. A methyl group given away by SAMe helps eliminate histamine from the body. Those with allergies or rashes may have higher levels of histamine and decreased methyl groups which produce a key component for your cell membranes called phosphatidylcholine. The methyl group donated by SAMe helps build phosphatidylcholine which then gets incorporated into the walls of all your cells, known as cell membranes. If these cell membranes become damaged and weak, the cells become fragile, allow toxins and harmful things into the cell, do not carry in useful nutrients and then they die. Excessive cell membrane damage can lead to serious medical conditions such as multiple sclerosis and cancer to name a few.[xvii]

SAMe®[xviii] IS THE BEST OPTION FOR 98% KIDS WITH ASD

SAMe is a naturally occurring metabolite found in the human body as well as in plant and animal foods. It is the most active of all methyl donors and has been compared to ATP in its importance for the body. SAMe is naturally synthesized in humans from the amino acid methionine in the presence of the cofactors B12 and folate.

SAMe is involved in the synthesis of neurotransmitters, the hormone melatonin, phospholipids, and polyamines, which control cellular growth. It is also the source of methyl groups inside the nucleus for DNA methylation, which controls gene expression and masking of genetic damage.

Try to get capsules that provide 200 mg of SAMe along with vitamins B6, B12, and folate as 5-MTHF in order to provide cofactors for the natural conversions of SAMe to L-homocysteine and then safely to L-cysteine.

MORE ON MTHFR

"The most common MTHFR mutation is called the MTHFR C677T mutation, or the "thermolabile" MTHFR mutation. Another common mutation is called MTHFR A1298C. To have any detrimental effect, mutations must be present in both copies of a person's MTHFR genes. Having only one mutation, ie, being heterozygous, is, from a medical perspective, irrelevant. Even when 2 MTHFR mutations are present (eg, 2 C677T mutations, or one C677T mutation and one A1298C mutation), not all people will develop high homocysteine levels. Although these mutations do impair the regulation of homocysteine, adequate folate levels essentially "cancel out" this defect."[xix]

Again in my #1 book, THE 85% SOLUTION, I detail this disease and how you should properly arrive at the diagnosis and treat it.

But regardless you start with an intracellular Spectracell™ Comprehensive Micronutrient Panel as young as they can go – 10? 11?

As I like to say this will guide you like footprints in the snow in order to decide if you need fairly inexpensive gene testing (I like SpectraCell™'s testing for MTHFR currently).

To summarize (again this is from THE 85% SOLUTION):

PROTOCOL FOR MTHFR

- o Start with seeing your doctor – make sure he understands biochemistry regarding MTHFR. Lay out your symptoms and what you think.

- o Start with a 1) SpectraCell™ Comprehensive Micronutrient Panel, 2) Homocysteine Level, 3) Whole Blood Histamine Level.

- o If your Spectracell Metabolic panel suggests you need it cover any other vitamins.

- o If suggestive on the Metabolic Panel (when it returns) then get the Spectracell™ MTHFR testing done and 23andme™ done too.

- o Look at your WHOLE BLOOD HISTAMINE LEVEL – you need to know your status – remember to have it drawn when they first check your Homocysteine level.

- ○ (REMEMBER -- if Whole Blood Histamine is LOW, the individual will be overmethylated. And if it is HIGH, they will be undermethylated.)

- ○ ★(FOR KIDS WITH ASD) Undermethylator (High Whole Blood Histamine Level >70 ng/ml) – SAMe works for these! Makes them happy! But don't give folate/folic acid! Also antidepressant SSRIs tend to work well with these people. Add SAMe at 400 mg a day – watch for depression or anxiety. My preferred brand is the <u>Source Naturals™ brand off Amazon at 400 mg of SAMe for 60 tablets</u>. One per day is usually sufficient.

- ○ Overmethylator (Low Histamine Level <40 ng/ml) – SAMe makes suicidal – DO NOT GIVE/TAKE! Give/take folate or folinic acid instead. Plus SSRI's are bad for these people. (NOT FOR KIDS WITH ASD).

- ○ So add MethylFolate (L-5-MTHF) or add SAMe according to your histamine status.

- ○ Repeat all three tests above on a regular basis.

CHAPTER THREE

MITOCHONDRIAL DYSFUNCTION

Another Root Cause Defect – Defining Mitochondrial Dysfunction

Now that we've defined the main duties of the mitochondrial what is Mitochondrial Dysfunction and why is it important in kids with ASD?

Mitochondrial Dysfunction or Mitochondrial Diseases result from failures of the mitochondria, specialized compartments present in every cell of the body except red blood cells. Mitochondria are responsible for creating more than 90% of the energy needed by the body to sustain life and support growth. When they fail, less and less energy is generated within the cell. Cell injury and even cell death follow. If this process is repeated throughout the body, whole systems begin to fail, and the life of the person in whom this is happening is severely compromised. The disease primarily affects children, but adult onset is becoming more and more common.

Diseases of the mitochondria appear to cause the most damage to cells of the brain, heart, liver, skeletal muscles, kidney and the endocrine and respiratory systems.

Depending on which cells are affected, symptoms may include loss of motor control, muscle weakness and pain, gastro-intestinal disorders and swallowing difficulties, poor growth, cardiac disease, liver disease, diabetes, respiratory complications, seizures, visual/hearing problems, lactic acidosis, developmental delays and susceptibility to infection.[xx]

Defining Mitochondrial Disease

Mitochondrial diseases are the result of either inherited (always from the mom) or spontaneous mutations in mtDNA or nDNA which lead to altered functions of the proteins or RNA molecules that normally reside in mitochondria. Problems with mitochondrial function, however, may only affect certain tissues as a result of factors occurring during development and growth that we do not yet understand. Even when tissue-specific isoforms of mitochondrial proteins are considered, it is difficult to explain the variable patterns of affected organ systems in the mitochondrial disease syndromes seen clinically.[xxi]

Genocopies of Mitochondrial Disease

Because mitochondria perform so many different functions in different tissues, there are literally hundreds of different mitochondrial diseases. Each disorder produces a spectrum of abnormalities that can be confusing to both patients and physicians in early stages of diagnosis. Because of the complex interplay between the hundreds of genes and cells that must cooperate to keep our metabolic machinery running smoothly, it is a hallmark of mitochondrial diseases that identical mtDNA mutations may not produce identical diseases. Genocopies are diseases that are caused by the same mutation but may not look the same clinically.[xxii]

The very nature of the mitochondrial diseases and their differences are what has made pinning this base problem of autism down and added to the confusion over the years.

Defective Mitochondria are disastrous for cell, body and toxin removal health!!

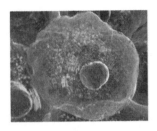 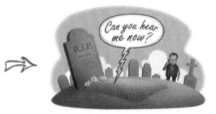

WAIT – Holy Cow! How Long Has This Been Known?
When Was Mitochondrial Disease First Recognized As The Root Cause Of ASD?

We've actually had an idea that Mitochondrial Dysfunction was a cause since 1998.

Med Hypotheses. 1998 Jun;50(6):497-500.

Autism: a mitochondrial disorder?

Lombard J[1].

Author information

[1]Westchester Square Medical Center, New York, NY 10461, USA.

Abstract

Autism is a developmental disorder characterized by disturbance in language, perception and socialization. A variety of biochemical, anatomical and neuroradiographical studies imply a disturbance of brain energy metabolism in autistic patients. The underlying etiology of a disturbed bioenergetic metabolism in autism is unknown. A likely etiological possibility may involve mitochondrial dysfunction with concomitant defects in neuronal oxidative phosphorylation within the central nervous system. This hypothesis is supported by a frequent association of lactic acidosis and carnitine deficiency in autistic patients. Mitochondria are vulnerable to a wide array of endogenous and exogenous factors which appear to be linked by excessive nitric oxide production. Strategies to augment mitochondrial function, either by decreasing production of endogenous toxic metabolites, reducing nitric oxide production, or stimulating mitochondrial enzyme activity may be beneficial in the treatment of autism.

PMID: 9710323 [PubMed - indexed for MEDLINE]

But who is Lombard J the author?

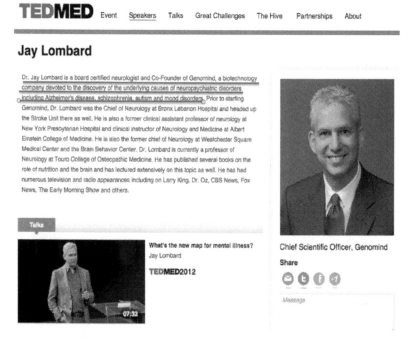

TEDMED Event Speakers Talks Great Challenges The Hive Partnerships About

Jay Lombard

Dr. Jay Lombard is a board certified neurologist and Co-Founder of Genomind, a biotechnology company devoted to the discovery of the underlying causes of neuropsychiatric disorders including Alzheimer's disease, schizophrenia, autism and mood disorders. Prior to starting Genomind, Dr. Lombard was the Chief of Neurology at Bronx Lebanon Hospital and headed up the Stroke Unit there as well. He is also a former clinical assistant professor of neurology at New York Presbyterian Hospital and clinical instructor of Neurology and Medicine at Albert Einstein College of Medicine. He is also the former chief of Neurology at Westchester Square Medical Center and the Brain Behavior Center. Dr. Lombard is currently a professor of Neurology at Touro College of Osteopathic Medicine. He has published several books on the role of nutrition and the brain and has lectured extensively on this topic as well. He has had numerous television and radio appearances including on Larry King, Dr. Oz, CBS News, Fox News, The Early Morning Show and others.

Talks

What's the new map for mental illness?
Jay Lombard
TEDMED2012

07:32

Chief Scientific Officer, Genomind

Share

Message

Kudos! Does he possibly deserve a Nobel Prize in Medicine?

For those parents of kids with autism or ASD, maybe he does.

That was 1998, What About Today?

Dr Lombard has been proven to be quite correct in his hypothesis.) The guy is a brilliant and curious man – kind of doctor I LOVE! Wow! Cool!)

Look at the following abstracts which all prove out what he said.

This 2011 review article points at the similarities in ASD and Mitochondrial Dysfunction.

Mitochondrial Disease and Autism

Pediatr Res. 2011 May;69(5 Pt 2):41R-7R. doi: 10.1203/PDR.0b013e318212f16b.

Mitochondrial dysfunction can connect the diverse medical symptoms associated with autism spectrum disorders.

Frye RE[1], Rossignol DA.

⊕ Author information

Abstract

Autism spectrum disorder (ASD) is a devastating neurodevelopmental disorder. Over the past decade, evidence has emerged that some children with ASD suffer from undiagnosed comorbid medical conditions. One of the medical disorders that has been consistently associated with ASD is mitochondrial dysfunction. Individuals with mitochondrial disorders without concomitant ASD manifest dysfunction in multiple high-energy organ systems, such as the central nervous, muscular, and gastrointestinal (GI) systems. Interestingly, these are the identical organ systems affected in a significant number of children with ASD. This finding increases the possibility that mitochondrial dysfunction may be one of the keys that explains the many diverse symptoms observed in some children with ASD. This article will review the importance of mitochondria in human health and disease, the evidence for mitochondrial dysfunction in ASD, the potential role of mitochondrial dysfunction in the comorbid medical conditions associated with ASD, and how mitochondrial dysfunction can bridge the gap for understanding how these seemingly disparate medical conditions are related. We also review the limitations of this evidence and other possible explanations for these findings. This new understanding of ASD should provide researchers a pathway for understanding the etiopathogenesis of ASD and clinicians the potential to develop medical therapies.

The next study discusses the panoply of differing levels of autism in the ASD – probably why it's called Autism SPECTRUM Disorder. In this study though they used CoQ10 (at it's base an anti-oxidant), L-carnitine (an amino acid which supports or increases testosterone) and B-vitamins (not sure why they did this) – the use of all of which led to improvements.

Mitochondrial Disease and ASD

Mol Psychiatry. 2012 Mar;17(3):290-314. doi: 10.1038/mp.2010.136. Epub 2011 Jan 25

Mitochondrial dysfunction in autism spectrum disorders: a systematic review and meta-analysis.

Rossignol DA[1], Frye RE.

@ Author information

Abstract

A comprehensive literature search was performed to collate evidence of mitochondrial dysfunction in autism spectrum disorders (ASDs) with two primary objectives. First, features of mitochondrial dysfunction in the general population of children with ASD were identified. Second, characteristics of mitochondrial dysfunction in children with ASD and concomitant mitochondrial disease (MD) were compared with published literature of two general populations: ASD children without MD, and non-ASD children with MD. The prevalence of MD in the general population of ASD was 5.0% (95% confidence interval 3.2, 6.9%), much higher than found in the general population (≈ 0.01%). The prevalence of abnormal biomarker values of mitochondrial dysfunction was high in ASD, much higher than the prevalence of MD. Variances and mean values of many mitochondrial biomarkers (lactate, pyruvate, carnitine and ubiquinone) were significantly different between ASD and controls. Some markers correlated with ASD severity. Neuroimaging, in vitro and post-mortem brain studies were consistent with an elevated prevalence of mitochondrial dysfunction in ASD. Taken together, these findings suggest children with ASD have a spectrum of mitochondrial dysfunction of differing severity. Eighteen publications representing a total of 112 children with ASD and MD (ASD/MD) were identified. The prevalence of developmental regression (52%), seizures (41%), motor delay (51%), gastrointestinal abnormalities (74%), female gender (39%), and elevated lactate (78%) and pyruvate (45%) was significantly higher in ASD/MD compared with the general ASD population. The prevalence of many of these abnormalities was similar to the general population of children with MD, suggesting that ASD/MD represents a distinct subgroup of children with MD. Most ASD/MD cases (79%) were not associated with genetic abnormalities, raising the possibility of secondary mitochondrial dysfunction. Treatment studies for ASD/MD were limited, although improvements were noted in some studies with carnitine, co-enzyme Q10 and B-vitamins. Many studies suffered from limitations, including small sample sizes, referral or publication biases, and variability in protocols for selecting children for MD workup, collecting mitochondrial biomarkers and defining MD. Overall, this evidence supports the notion that mitochondrial dysfunction is associated with ASD. Additional studies are needed to further define the role of mitochondrial dysfunction in ASD.

The next study used neuropathologic studies (they performed on autopsy) looking at genetic levels of data in these ASD people. The very in depth study confirmed that genetic mutations in mitochondrial function were associated with ASD in these patients.

Mitochondrial Disease and ASD

Semin Pediatr Neurol. 2013 Sep;20(3):163-75. doi: 10.1016/j.spen.2013.10.008. Epub 2013 Oct 29.

Mitochondrial dysfunction in autism.

Legido A[1], Jethva R[2], Goldenthal MJ[2].

@ Author information

Abstract

Using data of the current prevalence of autism as 200:10,000 and a 1:2000 incidence of definite mitochondrial (mt) disease, if there was no linkage of autism spectrum disorder (ASD) and mt disease, it would be expected that 1 in 110 subjects with mt disease would have ASD and 1 in 2000 individuals with ASD would have mt disease. The co-occurrence of autism and mt disease is much higher than these figures, suggesting a possible pathogenetic relationship. Such hypothesis was initially suggested by the presence of biochemical markers of abnormal mt metabolic function in patients with ASD, including elevation of lactate, pyruvate, or alanine levels in blood, cerebrospinal fluid, or brain; carnitine level in plasma; and level of organic acids in urine, and by demonstrating impaired mt fatty acid β-oxidation. More recently, mtDNA genetic mutations or deletions or mutations of nuclear genes regulating mt function have been associated with ASD in patients or in neuropathologic studies on the brains of patients with autism. In addition, the presence of dysfunction of the complexes of the mt respiratory chain or electron transport chain, indicating abnormal oxidative phosphorylation, has been reported in patients with ASD and in the autopsy samples of brains. Possible pathogenetic mechanisms linking mt dysfunction and ASD include mt activation of the immune system, abnormal mt $Ca(2+)$ handling, and mt-induced oxidative stress. Genetic and epigenetic regulation of brain development may also be disrupted by mt dysfunction, including mt-induced oxidative stress. The role of the purinergic system linking mt dysfunction and ASD is currently under investigation. In summary, there is genetic and biochemical evidence for a mitochondria (mt) role in the pathogenesis of ASD in a subset of children. To determine the prevalence and type of genetic and biochemical mt defects in ASD, there is a need for further research using the latest genetic technology such as next-generation sequencing, microarrays, bioinformatics, and biochemical assays. Because of the availability of potential therapeutic options for mt disease, successful research results could translate into better treatment and outcome for patients with mt-associated ASD. This requires a high index of suspicion of mt disease in children with autism who are diagnosed early.

© 2013 Published by Elsevier Inc.

Transl Psychiatry. 2013 Jun 18;3:e273. doi: 10.1038/tp.2013.51.

Redox metabolism abnormalities in autistic children associated with mitochondrial disease.

Frye RE[1], Delatorre R, Taylor H, Slattery J, Melnyk S, Chowdhury N, James SJ.

@ Author information

Abstract

Research studies have uncovered several metabolic abnormalities associated with autism spectrum disorder (ASD), including mitochondrial disease (MD) and abnormal redox metabolism. Despite the close connection between mitochondrial dysfunction and oxidative stress, the relation between MD and oxidative stress in children with ASD has not been studied. Plasma markers of oxidative stress and measures of cognitive and language development and ASD behavior were obtained from 18 children diagnosed with ASD who met criteria for probable or definite MD per the Morava et al. criteria (ASD/MD) and 18 age and gender-matched ASD children without any biological markers or symptoms of MD (ASD/NoMD). Plasma measures of redox metabolism included reduced free glutathione (fGSH), oxidized glutathione (GSSG), the fGSH/GSSG ratio and 3-nitrotyrosine (3NT). In addition, a plasma measure of chronic immune activation, 3-chlorotyrosine (3CT), was also measured. Language was measured using the preschool language scale or the expressive one-word vocabulary test (depending on the age), adaptive behaviour was measured using the Vineland Adaptive Behavior Scale (VABS) and core autism symptoms were measured using the Autism Symptoms Questionnaire and the Social Responsiveness Scale. Children with ASD/MD were found to have lower scores on the

certain supplements, the use of such supplements were not found to be related to the redox biomarkers that were related to cognitive development or behavior in the ASD/MD group but could possibly account for the difference in glutathione metabolism noted between groups. This study suggests that different subgroups of children with ASD have different redox abnormalities, which may arise from different sources. A better understanding of the relationship between mitochondrial dysfunction in ASD and oxidative stress, along with other factors that may contribute to oxidative stress, will be critical to understanding how to guide treatment and management of ASD children. This study also suggests that it is important to identify ASD/MD children as they may respond differently to specific treatments because of their specific metabolic profile.

This study showed that the causes of ASD are indeed multifactorial but that oxidative stress was a predominant issue or effect of the autism (we'll get more into this later in treatment options). Though they do not define the exact oxidative stress or defect associated with autism (another point we'll develop later in detail).

CHAPTER 4

CAUSES OF MITOCHONDRIAL DYSFUNCTION MUTATIONS IN CHILDREN

Remember this – "Mitochondrial diseases are the result of either inherited or spontaneous mutations in mtDNA or nDNA which lead to altered functions of the proteins or RNA molecules that normally reside in mitochondria."

So are there known causes of spontaneous mutations in mtDNA or nDNA that can be addressed or prevented so we can stop this wave of autistic children or at least slow it?

Possibly…

Remember, Mitochondrial Dysfunction causes:

- Alack of ATP (basic energy)
- Damaged cells cannot go through cell death (no apoptosis)
- Toxins are not properly removed from system
- Loss of motor control
- Weakness and Fatigue
- Poor growth
- Seizures
- Liver disease
- Visual Problems
- Hearing Problems
- and more!

But what can cause this permanent dysfunction of the mitochondria at a genetic level in a human being?

Can MTHFR Gene Mutation Cause Mitochondrial Dysfunction?

Yes.

If you have an issue with your MTHFR gene, and for that matter any other gene in your methylation cycle – it will have a downstream effect on your mitochondria. And it is known folate conversion also affects glutathione production, and it has been shown in other studies that mitochondrial dysfunction patients (and autistic children) are low in glutathione, meaning that their ability to detoxify certain environmental stressors (such as chemicals, food additives, bacteria and medications) is low, meaning that these stressors can cause more damage the longer they hang around inside the body and the cell- especially to your mitochondria. So MTHFR GENE MUTATION = LOW INTRACELLULAR FOLATE (B12) = LOW GLUTATHIONE PRODUCTION = LOW DETOXIFICATION = HIGHER TOXIC LOAD = MORE MITOCHONDRIAL DAMAGE = MORE GENE MUTATIONS.

Got it?

This diagram may help further (MTHFR is in the center) and how blocking THF (Tetra-Hydra-Folate) causes a BIG problem with the Krebs Cycle and the mitochondria and glutathione production.

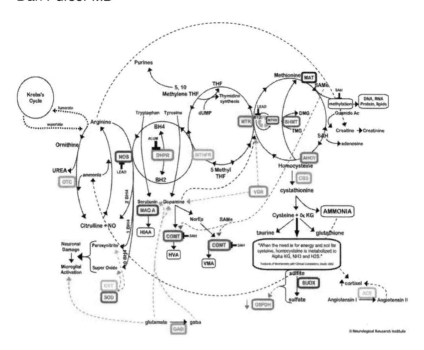

Can Vitamin D3 Levels Cause a Problem Too?

Vitamin D3 from a mom's perspective?

Acta Psychiatr Scand. 2011 May;123(5):339-48. doi: 10.1111/j.1600-0447.2010.01662.x. Epub 2011 Jan 11.

Prevalence of autism according to maternal immigrant status and ethnic origin.

Dealberto MJ.

ⓘ Author information

Abstract

OBJECTIVE: To examine the rates of autism separately according to maternal immigrant status and ethnic origin in respect to the vitamin D insufficiency hypothesis.

METHOD: Articles were identified by electronic searches. Studies were selected when they analysed autism rates according to maternal immigrant status and/or ethnic origin using multivariate techniques.

RESULTS: This review gave further support to the association between maternal immigrant status and an increased risk of autism. The relationship with ethnic origin was more complex. Although the crude rates did not differ, multivariate analyses taking into account confounding factors found that black ethnicity was associated with an increased risk for autism. The risk was highly significant when considering the strict definition of autistic disorders as opposed to the large definition of other pervasive developmental disorders. The risk was also very significant for autism associated with mental retardation.

CONCLUSION: These results are consistent with the maternal vitamin D insufficiency hypothesis. Neurobiological studies are warranted to document the effect of maternal vitamin D insufficiency during pregnancy on the foetal brain and the window of vulnerability. This review stresses the importance of monitoring vitamin D levels in pregnant women, especially those who are immigrant, dark-skinned or veiled, and the urgency of randomized controlled trials.

Low Vitamin D levels in the mother during pregnancy in 2011 (in this study these were immigrant mothers but that's actually not important since we're all descended from immigrants anyway...).

But here's a newer 2014 study that explains more.

Vitamin D3 and ASD/Autism

FASEB J. 2014 Feb 20. [Epub ahead of print]

Vitamin D hormone regulates serotonin synthesis. Part 1: relevance for autism.

Patrick RP[1], Ames BN.

⊛ Author information

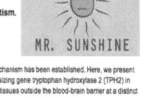

MR. SUNSHINE

Abstract

Serotonin and vitamin D have been proposed to play a role in autism; however, no causal mechanism has been established. Here, we present evidence that vitamin D hormone (calcitriol) activates the transcription of the serotonin-synthesizing gene tryptophan hydroxylase 2 (TPH2) in the brain at a vitamin D response element (VDRE) and represses the transcription of TPH1 in tissues outside the blood-brain barrier at a distinct VDRE. The proposed mechanism explains 4 major characteristics associated with autism: the low concentrations of serotonin in the brain and its elevated concentrations in tissues outside the blood-brain barrier; the low concentrations of the vitamin D hormone precursor 25-hydroxyvitamin D [25(OH)D$_3$]; the high male prevalence of autism; and the presence of maternal antibodies against fetal brain tissue. Two peptide hormones, oxytocin and vasopressin, are also associated with autism and genes encoding the oxytocin-neurophysin I preproprotein, the oxytocin receptor, and the arginine vasopressin receptor contain VDREs for activation. Supplementation with vitamin D and tryptophan is a practical and affordable solution to help prevent autism and possibly ameliorate some symptoms of the disorder.-Patrick, R. P., Ames, B. N. Vitamin D hormone regulates serotonin synthesis. Part 1: relevance for autism.

Read about the "4 MAJOR characteristics" associated with autism in this study, especially maternal antibodies to fetal brain tissue cause by low maternal Vitamin D3 levels. Are these antibodies attacking the mitochondria the cause of the mitochondrial dysfunction?

In my particular practice I check intracellular levels of D3 often (more about this later) and in cold snowy Utah find low D3 levels to be quite common – probably the most common vitamin deficiency I see. And it's possibly associated with ASD causally? Are you kidding me?

Are there other maternal vitamin deficiencies associated with causing lack of neurological development in neonates?

The answer turns out to be yes.

What is DHA? Helps with Child IQ

Am J Clin Nutr. 2013 Dec;98(6):1575-82. doi: 10.3945/ajcn.112.051524. Epub 2013 Sep 25.

Maternal fatty acids in pregnancy, FADS polymorphisms, and child intelligence quotient at 8 y of age.

Steer CD[1], Lattka E, Koletzko B, Golding J, Hibbeln JR.

@ Author information

Abstract

BACKGROUND: Brain tissue is selectively enriched with highly unsaturated fatty acids (FAs). Altering the maternal FA status in pregnancy may improve fetal neural development with lasting consequences for child development.

OBJECTIVE: We explored whether maternal FAs in erythrocytes, either measured directly or indirectly by maternal FADS genetic variants, are associated with child intelligence quotient (IQ).

DESIGN: Linear regression analyses, adjusted for 18 confounders, were used to investigate the associations in 2839 mother-child pairs from the population-based Avon Longitudinal Study of Parents and Children cohort.

RESULTS: Low levels of arachidonic acid (20:4n-6) were associated with lower performance IQ (-2.0 points; 95% CI: -3.5, -0.6 points; P = 0.007, increased R^2 = 0.27%), high levels of osbond acid (22:5n-6) were associated with verbal IQ (-1.8 points; 95% CI: -3.2, -0.4 points; P = 0.014, R^2 = 0.20%), and high levels of adrenic acid (22:4n-6) were associated with verbal IQ (-1.7 points; 95% CI:-3.1, -0.3 points; P = 0.016, R^2 = 0.19%). There was some evidence to support a negative association of low docosahexaenoic acid (DHA; 22:6n-3) with full-scale IQ (R^2 = 0.15%). Novel weak associations were also observed for low levels of osbond acid (R^2 ≤ 0.29%) and FADS variants with opposite effects for intron variants and variants in the promoter region such as rs3834458 (R^2 ≤ 0.38%).

CONCLUSIONS: These results support the positive role of maternal arachidonic acid and DHA on fetal neural development, although the effects on child IQ by 8 y of age were small (0.1 SD), with other factors contributing more substantially. The endogenous synthesis of these FAs by FADS genes, especially FADS2, may also be important. The replication of these results is recommended.

DHA is the best, most helpful (physiologically and nootropically) part of fish oil (the other being EPA).

Turns out pregnant moms need lots of it too – so they have neurologically healthy children later.

CHAPTER 5

BUT WHAT ABOUT THINGS MOMS TAKE DURING PREGNANCY?

There has been one association in modern medicine that's interesting.

If women take SSRI's (such as fluoxetine, etc.)

during pregnancy there's been an association with autism, but the causality remains to be confirmed (and this was a BIG retrospective study where they were looking hard at SSRIs).

Neurosci Biobehav Rev. 2015 Feb;49:82-9. doi: 10.1016/j.neubiorev.2014.11.020. Epub 2014 Dec 9.

Exposure to selective serotonin reuptake inhibitors during pregnancy and risk of autism spectrum disorder in children: a systematic review and meta-analysis of observational studies.

Man KK[1], Tong HH[2], Wong LY[1], Chan EW[1], Simonoff E[3], Wong IC[4].

⊕ Author information

Abstract

This study is a critical analysis of the association between selective serotonin reuptake inhibitors (SSRIs) exposure during pregnancy and autism spectrum disorder (ASD) risk in children. Electronic databases were searched for observational studies published from January 1946 to June 2014 related to the association between SSRI exposure during pregnancy and ASD in children. Studies relevant to the association between SSRI exposure during pregnancy and ASD in children were extracted and compiled for meta-analysis evaluation. Ninety-five citations were identified and seven observational studies were included. Four case-control studies were eligible for the meta-analysis and two cohort studies were narratively reviewed. The pooled crude and adjusted odds ratios of the case-control studies were 2.13 (95% CI 1.66-2.73) and 1.81 (95% CI 1.47-2.24) respectively. Low heterogeneity was observed between studies. The two population-based cohort studies, utilizing the same Denmark data set, have conflicting results. The findings of this meta-analysis and narrative review support an increased risk of ASD in children of mothers exposed to SSRIs during pregnancy; however, the causality remains to be confirmed.

Copyright © 2014 Elsevier Ltd. All rights reserved.

If it were my wife or me (if I was female) – I'd stop taking them and use another option if I was pregnant.

CHAPTER 6

INSTEAD OF BLAMING US MOMS, ARE THERE VITAMINS WE SHOULD BE GIVING OUR KIDS?

Yes, studies have shown there are several that benefit ASD kids.

And logic, knowledge of the marketplace, and reasoning tells me there might be one more HUGE one out there that could help.

The research is SCANT -- there's just little of it. It's

weird. I assumed there would be tons of it but there's actually not. I was shocked as I looked at and for studies on ASD and supplements. Not sure where all the money's going to for ASD research – but it's not being used on vitamins for the public. Probably going to drug company research.

So let's look at the vitamins and the studies out there.

DocosaHexaenoic Acid (DHA)
DHA is the best part of fish oil.

DHA levels in the pregnant mother is critical to the intelligence (IQ) of the child and probably impacts autism somewhat.[xxiii]

Lack of DHA (LCPUFA) in another study with maternal levels showed that hyperactivity and schizophrenia were at a higher risk in mother's who had a DHA deficiency occurring.[xxiv]

But in the most recent study and one directly involving young adults with severe autism, DHA supplementation was not found to help either way.[xxv]

If I had a child with autism or ASD would I still use it? Yes.

CoQ10 (Ubiqionol)

CoQ10 is the ultimate Kreb's cycle participant. Without COQ10 you get really fatigued (sound familiar?) and brain fogged – I do enough intracellular testing and treatment of patients that I've seen this numerous times. Imagine if this was your daily existence? It'd be horrible.

I prefer the ubiquinol form of CoQ10 due to it's increased bioavailability but I don't really think it matters. A typical dose is 200 mg a day.

"Manipulated B Vitamins"

These very specific B vitamins are for the homozygous or worse MTHFR cases but make sure you have intracellular vitamin testing then genetic testing done before you let them start on these vitamins (both available through Spectracell™) – those tests give you what I call footprints in the snow to follow to so you can get the child on the correct B vitamin.

There are certain "manipulated vitamins" that have been designed to work around the MTHFR mutations – they are called L-5-MTHF™ and Homocysteine Supreme™ and SAM-E™. Designed to prevent over-methylation, they are very effective. But be careful, you must take the version compatible with your mutation – mainly SAM-E or SAMe since 98% of people with ASD are undermethylators.

These are physician prescribed (and sold) vitamins and they need to be prescribed by a knowledgeable physician who understands MTHFR and has ordered all the tests and knows how to use them properly.

Brain Nootropics

Nootropics (the term brain nootropic is a little redundant but works for this situation), also referred to as smart drugs, memory enhancers, neuro enhancers, cognitive enhancers, and intelligence enhancers, are drugs, supplements, nutraceuticals, and functional foods that improve one or more aspects of mental function, such as working memory, motivation, and attention[xxvi].

Alpha-Lipoic Acid (ALA)

Lipoic acid is cofactor for at least five enzyme systems. Two of these are in the citric acid cycle through which many organisms turn nutrients into energy and this book has so far been, at it's core, about the citric acid (Kreb's) cycle and how it's damage effects kid's brains and causes autism.

Think of ALA as another CoQ10 -- it's that important -- it's also a critical part of the Kreb's cycle.

Researched Benefits:

• ALA may lower inflammation

• ALA is neuroprotective against Alzheimer's Disease

- ALA helps against viral induced Central Nervous System-induced pathologies

Not surprisingly (okay, it surprises me but really should it at this point?) there have been no studies regarding ALA benefiting ASD.

Alpha-GPC (L-Alpha Glycerylphosphoryl Choline)

L-Alpha glycerylphosphorylcholine (alpha-GPC, choline alfoscerate) is a natural choline compound found in the brain. It is also a parasympathomimetic acetylcholine precursor[xxvii] which may have potential for the treatment of Alzheimer's disease and dementia.[xxviii]

Alpha-GPC rapidly delivers choline to the brain across the blood–brain barrier and is a biosynthetic precursor of the acetylcholine neurotransmitter.[xxix] It is a non-prescription drug in most countries and in the United States it is classified as generally recognized as safe (GRAS).[xxx]

Bizarrely there's only one study with ASD (and it's not even actually Alpha-GPC they use). But it did work -- giving some noticeable benefits in combination therapy with other nootropics.[xxxi]

Phosphatidyl Serine (PS)

Phosphatidyl Serine is another nootropic whose time has come with ASD.

There have been no studies done though – something I find very odd.

I cannot understand this but it seems to be a repeat problem. Probably there is no big pharma so no funding to do the study. Maybe some pediatric university hospital could fund it.

Acetyl-L-Carnitine (ALCAR)

ALCAR is an amino acid that's been used to help with improving sperm count and testosterone production.

L-carnitine is a derivative of the amino acid, lysine. In healthy people, carnitine homeostasis (balance) is maintained through endogenous biosynthesis of L-carnitine, absorption of carnitine from dietary sources, and elimination and reabsorption of carnitine by the kidneys.[xxxii]

Bioavailability of ALCAR is thought to be higher than L-carnitine.

L-carnitine is synthesized primarily in the liver but also in the kidneys and then transported to other tissues. It is most concentrated in tissues that use fatty acids as their primary fuel, such as skeletal and cardiac (heart) muscle. In this regard, L-carnitine plays an important role in energy production by conjugating fatty acids for transport into the mitochondria.

L-carnitine is required for mitochondrial beta-oxidation of long-chain fatty acids for energy production.

It's also thought to help with memory and brain health.[xxxiii]

But more importantly it has shown benefits to ASD.

GLUTATHIONE

Glutathione is the ultimate anti-oxidant -- the master anti-oxidant as the job of all other anti-oxidants, such as Vitamin C, is to absorb the oxidant or toxin from the glutathione molecule, in order to reduce it. So all other anti-oxidants serve the glutathione molecule.

The glutathione molecule has a very sticky end or tip (and stinky, as this is what gives it it's distinct smell) so that it will attach to anything perceived as foreign to the human body -- this is the SH or sulfhydryl group. Glutathione's main job (with it's sticky end protruding out) is to sit on top of a T-killer white blood cell (such as a CD4 or CD8) and the white blood cell uses the sticky end of the GSH since it appears to be designed to spear and carry off (spearing is actually called "conjugation" and the carrying is termed "transport") and toxins or metals or anti-oxidants -- this is fairly analogous to how a porcupine uses quills to scare away or spear enemies.

NAC vs GSH

NAC is considered to be the ain (usually missing or later). N-Acetyl-Cysteine is an amino acid – it's also the most important (since it's always low in a LOT of humans) precursor to glutathione.

Lack of NAC is usually not the problem in kids with ASD – it's the inability to convert GSSG back to GSH.

You can still give ASD children NAC – it comes in 600 mg and you take it twice a day but just know because of the side effects (nausea mostly) I would give younger kids one a day and only maybe for a 100 days every year. Stop it after the bottle is gone.

And watch for side effects as they do exist.

TRUTHS & RULES ABOUT GLUTATHIONE:

Glutathione is tri-peptide (meaning it's made of three conjoined amino acids) and if you give it orally it will be at least digested to its three amino acid components.

Since that seems to be a major point of misunderstanding with glutathione let me say it again but differently: you can take it topically or intravenously -- really those are your only options.

Glutathione is relatively hard for human bodies to create – and harder yet to keep in reduced form.

Reduced form (GSH) is the best most powerful option.

GSH cannot be kept stable against oxidization unless it's protected somehow -- the how has been the question.

We have done much research in this area and do have a reduced and stable GSH that's topical (remember it cannot be oral) that we complexed to a carbohydrate to protect it from the oxygen in the air – just spray it on and instant absorption – it has been extremely promising and though considered GRAS-E by the FDA, we are currently going through the FDA approval process so we can make the appropriate claims.

Essential Oils

Citrus Oils contain D-Limonene, which increases de novo glutathione production in the liver.

Orange Oil increased GSH 70% in the study I performed

The highest concentration of d-limonene in any essential oil is Grapefruit but it remains unusable for topical use as it will burn the skin.

Orange or Lime essential oils are mellow, won't burn your skin, and work very well to increase glutathione levels in normal adults. Just beware however that they will turn your skin black (like a tattoo just not as permanent).

Beware Potential Toxicity

But toxicity is a consideration as d-limonene can build up and cause liver toxicity in kids with ASD. This is a problem and speaks as to the real cause for low GSH levels in kids with ASD -- they do not create enough GPX so they can't reduce GSSG (GSSG or the oxidized form of glutathione) to GSH (the reduced form).

PQQ (Pyrroquinoline Quinone)

Discovered in the 1960's this vitamin is making it's big surge as we speak. Just think of it as the ultimate mitochondrial support out there.

KEY POINTS:

Another form of CoQ10 but for the brain and supports the mitochondria

PQQ has huge FDA validated benefits:

- Stimulates formation of mitochondria in the liver
- PQQ aids in mitochondrial function
- PQQ protects the mitochondria against oxidative stress
- PQQ rescues neurons
- PQQ protects against neurotrauma
- PQQ protects against mercury toxicity
- PQQ protects better than SOD
- PQQ up-regulates mitochondrial genes in the face of ROS insults
- PQQ causes mitochondrial biogenesis especially in neurons
- PQQ improves memory 30% after six weeks of taking it in one validated study (by the FDA) in patients with dementia or memory loss.
- Need to take it with CoQ10 to get these benefits.
- No PQQ studies with ASD have been done but they clearly should be -- if I had funding I would do this.

My complaint is if ASD is from mitochondrial disease then why haven't any studies been done with PQQ and AUTISM. My argument to you is put your ASD child on this as it can't hurt and might be the piece that brings them back from the brink.

Dan Purser MD

CHAPTER 7

BUT WHAT ABOUT THINGS MOMS TAKE DURING PREGNANCY THAT COULD CAUSE HARM?

Okay, now I'm back to blaming moms (not really -- just teasing).

There has been one association in modern medicine that's interesting.

Fluoxetine has been shown in more than one study to cause genetic changes when introduced maternally or neonatally to unborn infants[xxxiv].

Do not take fluoxetine or SSRIs if you do not want this risk. Sorry if you have, too.

CHAPTER 8

TESTING I FIND USEFUL

1. Spectracell® Comprehensive Micronutrient Panel (www.spectracell.com)
2. Whole Blood Histamine Level
3. Homocysteine Level
4. 23andme.com DNA testing
5. Spectracell® MTHFR testing

CHAPTER 9

MY ASD PROTOCOL

Make sure you get a Spectracell Comprehensive Micronutrient Panel – this is where you dive deep right up front. Go to www.spectracell.com to find a doctor near you who offers this test. Pay cash if you need to – just get it done.

If Micronutrient Panel shows B vitamin, zinc, magnesium, and/or glutathione deficiencies then be suspicious -- get a Spectracell MTHFR testing done next along with a Whole Blood Histamine and Homocysteine level. Also get 23andme testing too. Please check out my book – THE 85% SOLUTION and many of the excellent blogs and websites like MTHFR.net for more info as this could get fairly complicated.

Get your child on the correct vitamins for the noted Spectracell® deficiencies

Add one drop Orange essential oil topically each day

Add the following vitamins & nootropics [in doses appropriate to your child's age and weight – but always start each one at a lower dose and less frequent than advised to play it safe].

- o PS – Phosphatidyl Serine
- o Alpha-GPC -- L-Alpha glycerylphosphorylcholine
- o ALA – Alpha-Lipoic Acid
- o D3 – Vitamin D3 – be careful as this can get toxic so no more than 2,000 units per day or 2X RDA for a child.
- o DHA – best part of fish oil.
- o CoQ10 – I like Qunol liquid – easy to give.

- o SAM-E – or start with methionine at 500 mg a day or less. Be careful.
- o BioPQQ™ with CoQ10 (I prefer Qunol™®)

If possible add topical complexed glutathione spray – one-two sprays a day – hard to find it but worth it.

Be patient and be careful as this may take a few months. Though if improvement is going to occur then it will come slowly but you will notice it.

© Copyright by Dan Purser MD of DP Publishing, LLC

Thank You!

I know you chose to read this book from millions of options, and I really appreciate it. It really does mean a lot to me, and my team that you would read this book that will change your life. If you enjoyed this book, and believe it did help you, <u>please take a moment to leave a review on my Amazon page.</u>

I, Dan Purser MD, personally go over every single review, to make sure my books really are reaching out and helping you. Please help me help you, by leaving a review!

-- Dan Purser MD

Want to Connect with Dr. Purser?

For men's information on testosterone issues and their medical problems and a more thoughtful approach to men's problems: http://www.drpursernaturaltestosterone.com

For Dr. Purser's Amazon Author Page linking to all of his books (including his five #1 books): http://www.greatmedebooks.com

To get to know Dr. Purser better and to get his email newsletter (full of discounts and coupons and freebies): http://drpurser.com

For women's information on their health issues (PMS, migraines, endometriosis, menopause, thyroid, and osteoporosis) and a more thoughtful approach to those problems: http://drpursernaturaloptions.com

Facebook: Dan Purser MD

Twitter #danpursermd

Pinterest: Dan Purser MD

© Copyright by Dan Purser MD of DP Publishing, LLC

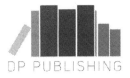

DP PUBLISHING

© Copyright 2015 by Dan Purser MD of Medutainment, Inc.

© Copyright 2015 by Dan Purser MD of Medutainment, Inc.

© Copyright 2015 by Dan Purser MD of Medutainment, Inc.

References

[i] No author listed. Accessed online 09 June 2015 at http://www.buzzle.com/articles/mitochondrial-function.html

[ii] Boris, M; Glodblatt, A. Association of MTHFR Gene Variants with Autism. Vol 9, No 4, Journal of the American Physicians and Surgeons, 2004. Accessed 1 August 2015 online at http://www.jpands.org/vol9no4/boris.pdf.

[iii] https://youtu.be/WMiOvYbFzgE

[iv] Tsafrir, J. Accessed online 17 June 2015 at http://primaldocs.com/members-blog/histamine-methylation-and-mthfr/

[v] Tsafrir, J. Accessed online 17 June 2015 at http://primaldocs.com/members-blog/histamine-methylation-and-mthfr/

[vi] Tsafrir, J. Accessed online 17 June 2015 at http://primaldocs.com/members-blog/histamine-methylation-and-mthfr/

[vii] Walsh, WJ. Accessed online 17 June 2015 at http://www.mensahmedical.com/images/Depression_PP_2.pdf

[viii] Walsh, WJ. Accessed online 17 June 2015 at http://www.mensahmedical.com/images/Depression_PP_2.pdf

[ix] Walsh, WJ. Accessed online 17 June 2015 at http://www.mensahmedical.com/images/Depression_PP_2.pdf

[x] Walsh, WJ. Accessed online 17 June 2015 at http://www.mensahmedical.com/images/Depression_PP_2.pdf

[xi] Walsh, WJ. Accessed online 17 June 2015 at http://www.mensahmedical.com/images/Depression_PP_2.pdf

[xii] Walsh, WJ. Accessed online 17 June 2015 at http://www.mensahmedical.com/images/Depression_PP_2.pdf

[xiii] Carnahan, J. Accessed online 17 June 2015 at http://doccarnahan.blogspot.com/2013/11/histamine-intolerance-could-this-be.html

[xiv] Tsafrir, J. Accessed online 17 June 2015 at http://primaldocs.com/members-blog/histamine-methylation-and-mthfr/

[xv] Tsafrir, J. Accessed online 17 June 2015 at http://primaldocs.com/members-blog/histamine-methylation-and-mthfr/

[xvi] No author listed. Accessed 12 May 2015 online at https://pgenpt.wordpress.com/2014/06/23/trying-out-sam-e-smart-people-can-do-dumb-things/

[xvii] SHOMON, M. Accessed 12 May 2015 online at http://thyroid.about.com/od/MTHFR-Gene-Mutations-and-Polymorphisms/fl/The-Link-Between-MTHFR-Gene-Mutations-and-Disease-Including-Thyroid-Health.htm

[xviii] No author listed. Accessed 13 May 2015 online at http://catalog.designsforhealth.com/SAMe

[xix] Varga, EA; Sturm, AC; Misita, CP; Moll, S; et al. Homocysteine and MTHFR Mutations, Relation to Thrombosis and Coronary Artery Disease, Accessed online 3 July 2015 at http://circ.ahajournals.org/content/111/19/e289.full

[xx] No author listed. Accessed online 09 June 2015 at http://www.umdf.org/site/c.8qKOJ0MvF7LUG/b.7934627/k.3711 /What_is_Mitochondrial_Disease.htm

[xxi] No author listed. Accessed online 09 June 2015 at http://www.umdf.org/site/c.8qKOJ0MvF7LUG/b.7934627/k.3711 /What_is_Mitochondrial_Disease.htm

[xxii] No author listed. Accessed online 09 June 2015 at http://www.umdf.org/site/c.8qKOJ0MvF7LUG/b.7934627/k.3711 /What_is_Mitochondrial_Disease.htm

[xxiii] Steer CD, Lattka E, et al. Maternal fatty acids in pregnancy, FADS polymorphisms, and child intelligence quotient at 8 y of age. Am J Clin Nutr. 2013 Dec;98(6):1575-82. doi: 10.3945/ajcn.112.051524

[xxiv] Janssen CI, Kiliaan AJ. Long-chain polyunsaturated fatty acids (LCPUFA) from genesis to senescence: the influence of LCPUFA on neural development, aging, and neurodegeneration. Prog Lipid Res. 2014 Jan;53:1-17. doi: 10.1016/j.plipres.2013.10.002.

[xxv] Politi P, Cena H, et al. Behavioral effects of omega-3 fatty acid supplementation in young adults with severe autism: an open label study. Arch Med Res. 2008 Oct;39(7):682-5. doi: 10.1016/j.arcmed.2008.06.005.

[xxvi] "Dorlands Medical Dictionary". Archived from the original on January 30, 2008.

[xxvii] De Jesus Moreno Moreno M (January 2003). "Cognitive improvement in mild to moderate Alzheimer's dementia after treatment with the acetylcholine precursor choline alfoscerate: a multicenter, double-blind, randomized, placebo-controlled trial". Clin Ther 25 (1): 178–93. doi:10.1016/S0149-2918(03)90023-3. PMID 12637119.

[xxviii] Doggrell SA & Evans S; Evans (October 2003). "Treatment of dementia with neurotransmission modulation". Expert Opin Investig Drugs 12 (10): 1633–1654. doi:10.1517/13543784.12.10.1633. PMID 14519085.

[xxix] Parnetti, Lucilla et al. (2007). "Cholinergic precursors in the treatment of cognitive impairment of vascular origin: Ineffective approaches or need for re-evaluation?". Journal of the Neurological Sciences 257 (1–2): 264–9. doi:10.1016/j.jns.2007.01.043. PMID 17331541.

© Copyright 2015 by Dan Purser MD of Medutainment, Inc.

[xxx] US Food and Drug Administration: Generally Recognized as Safe (GRAS) Determination for the Use of AlphaSize Alpha-Glycerylphosphoryl Choline.

[xxxi] Krasnoperova MG, Simashkova NV, Bashina VM. [Use of cholinomimetics in the treatment of endogenous autism in children]. [Article in Russian] Zh Nevrol Psikhiatr Im S S Korsakova. 2004;104(6):35-9.

[xxxii] No author listed. Accessed 17 July 2015 online at http://lpi.oregonstate.edu/mic/dietary-factors/L-carnitine

[xxxiii] No author listed. Accessed 17 July 2015 online at http://lpi.oregonstate.edu/mic/dietary-factors/L-carnitine

[xxxiv] Zimmerberg B, Germeyan SC. Effects of neonatal fluoxetine exposure on behavior across development in rats selectively bred for an infantile affective trait. Dev Psychobiol. 2015 Mar;57(2):141-52. doi: 10.1002/dev.21264.

Index

A

© Copyright 2015 by Dan Purser MD of Medutainment, Inc.

© Copyright 2015 by Dan Purser MD of Medutainment, Inc.

© Copyright 2015 by Dan Purser MD of Medutainment, Inc.

© Copyright 2015 by Dan Purser MD of Medutainment, Inc.

© Copyright 2015 by Dan Purser MD of Medutainment, Inc.

51026517R00052

Made in the USA
Lexington, KY
09 April 2016